UTILIZATION MANAGEMENT: A HANDBOOK FOR PSYCHIATRISTS

UTILIZATION MANAGEMENT: A HANDBOOK FOR PSYCHIATRISTS

The Committee on Managed Care
of the American Psychiatric Association

Published by the
American Psychiatric Association
1400 K Street, N.W.
Washington, DC 20005

Note: The contributors have worked to ensure that all information in this book concerning drug dosages, schedules, and routes of administration is accurate as of the time of publication and consistent with standards set by the U.S. Food and Drug Administration and the general medical community. As medical research and practice advance, however, therapeutic standards may change. For this reason and because human and mechanical errors sometimes occur, we recommend that readers follow the advice of a physician who is directly involved in their care or the care of a member of their family.

The findings, opinions, and conclusions of this report do not necessarily represent the views of officers, trustees, or all members of the American Psychiatric Association. This report represents the judgment and consensus of the experts who wrote it.

Copyright © 1992 American Psychiatric Association

ALL RIGHTS RESERVED

Manufactured in the United States of America on acid-free paper

95 94 93 92   6 5 4 3 2 1

Library of Congress Cataloging-in-Publication Data
Utilization Management: A Handbook for Psychiatrists / by The
  Committee on Managed Care of the American Psychiatric Association
      p. cm.
  Includes bibliographical references (p.   ).
  ISBN 0-89042-235-4

91-47117
CIP

British Library Cataloguing in Publication Data
A CIP record is available from the British Library.

CONTENTS

FOREWORD

The practice of psychiatry has been transformed by those who pay the bill. Concerns about the costs of medical care generally and psychiatric care in particular have moved third-party payers, both public and private, to actively review and regulate treatment. Managed care and utilization management as a part of managed care are ever-present realities for hospital- and office-based psychiatrists. Prior and concurrent review of care over the 800 telephone line is a dimension of treatment planning not included in traditional residency training. There is an urgent need for advising on the appropriate interaction and behavior on both ends of the telephone line.

This handbook, which represents the efforts of The Committee on Managed Care of the American Psychiatric Association, is an attempt to provide to clinicians timely and useful information that will improve a mutual adaptational process and expedite what is the goal of both clinician and reviewer: quality patient care. Because this is likely to go through several revisions, the committee would appreciate feedback from members on the content (send to Committee on Managed Care, American Psychiatric Association, 1400 K Street, N.W., Washington, DC 20005).

As the world moves from one era of cost containment to another, it is important that the profession continue to take a proactive role in regulating itself. The Committee on Managed Care, through this handbook, is trying to enhance this process.

Steven S. Sharfstein, M.D.
Chair, The Committee on Managed Care,
American Psychiatric Association

CHAPTER 1

INTRODUCTION

Utilization management is a set of techniques used by or on behalf of purchasers of health care benefits to manage health care costs by influencing patient care decision making through case-by-case assessments of the appropriateness of care prior to and during its provision (1). Utilization management originated in the health maintenance organization (HMO), community mental health, and Medicare Professional Standards Review Commissions and later peer review organization (PRO) initiatives. It spread into the private, fee-for-service insurance sector in the early 1980s, where it continues to grow, driven by payers' concerns with rising health care costs. Today, nearly 80% of all insured persons have some form of utilization management built into their insurance contracts, and that percentage continues to increase.

The proliferation of managed care renders knowledge of its operation essential for all psychiatrists. This handbook is intended to be a functional guide to assist psychiatrists in navigating the process of utilization management to obtain optimal coverage for their patients. The handbook is a nonpolicy and nontheoretical document. It is written as a basic reference to provide definitions and models and information on process and contracting in utilization management. Frequent problems and their solutions and issues of confidentiality are also addressed. Appendixes 1–4 include names and addresses of chief executive officers or medical directors of major managed care and utilization review companies and major health insurance companies, addresses of state insurance commissioners, and a selected managed care bibliography. Issues of legislation and regulation, health services research, maintenance of a clearinghouse for information on problems in utilization management, ethics, and dialogue with the industry are addressed in separate initiatives of the American Psychiatric Association.

MODELS OF UTILIZATION MANAGEMENT AND MANAGED CARE

A plethora of utilization management options have evolved because nearly all third-party payers offer or contract for utilization management services. Utilization management is practiced in both public and private insurance. It is provided by health maintenance organizations (HMOs), commercial insurers that offer or contract for utilization management in addition to their insurance services, Medicare peer review organizations (PROs), and state Medicaid agencies. Furthermore, there are independent utilization management organizations, including employee assistance programs (EAPs), utilization review companies, and other managed care organizations offering both utilization review and provider networks.

With variations and hybrid phenomena, three basic models now predominate: 1) utilization review only, 2) utilization review with a select provider network, and 3) financially at-risk, prepaid HMOs. All three models use utilization review. Only HMOs and managed care organizations create a network of providers. The HMO is financially at risk for the total cost of treatment as well as administration. The vendor offering utilization review alone or utilization review with a select provider network is at risk only for the administrative costs of the program. However, these entities have a significant interest in cost containment because the future of their contracts naturally depends on employer satisfaction with the cost-containment experience.

The trend in the utilization management industry is clearly toward development of managed care organizations offering both utilization review and provider networks and a full range of service and continuum of care. A lesser trend is for managed care organizations to assume financial risk for provision of care. Although the terms *utilization management* and *managed care* are sometimes used interchangeably, for the purpose of clarity, this handbook will use *utilization management* to denote the generic concept of case-by-case allocation of resources, whereas *managed care* will refer to the combination of utilization management with a select provider network. *Utilization review* is an element of utilization management and denotes the actual process of medical record evaluation.

As the models suggest, participation in utilization management assumes many forms. Indeed, all psychiatrists are involved in utilization management in at least one of these forms. Even physicians who have made no contractual agreements with utilization management or managed care organizations will be subject to outside utilization review specified in their patients' health insurance contracts or through their hospitals' own utilization monitoring system that is required by Joint Commission on Accreditation of Healthcare Organizations (JCAHO) accreditation and Medicare and Medicaid participation.

An increasing number of psychiatrists in fee-for-service practice contract with one or more select or "preferred" provider organizations (PPOs), agreeing to discounted fee schedules, participation in utilization review, and other administrative requirements of the managed care organization in exchange for patient referral and reduced administrative burdens. Patients are offered financial incentives to use the network and are usually subjected to higher copayments if they choose a nonnetwork provider. In HMOs, psychiatrists may be full- or part-time employees with capitation contracts or may agree to receive specialty referrals from the HMO based on negotiated fee schedules. Still other psychiatrists work for the managed care industry itself, providing utilization management of care, establishing and maintaining criteria for review, and sometimes delivering care to a defined group.

THE PROCESS OF UTILIZATION MANAGEMENT

The process of utilization management is inherent in its definition. Again, utilization management is a set of techniques used by or on behalf of purchasers of health care benefits to manage health care costs by influencing patient care decision making through case-by-case assessments of the appropriateness of care prior to and during its provision (1). Case-by-case assessment prior to the provision or continued provision of care drives the process of utilization management, which includes

- Prior review
- Concurrent review
- Discharge planning
- Case management
- Retrospective review

In health maintenance organizations (HMOs), utilization management is performed by a review committee within the HMO, whereas with fee-for-service insurance, utilization management is performed by an independent review entity.

REFERRAL

In most HMOs and in some select or "preferred" provider organizations (PPOs), referral to a psychiatrist must be made by a primary care physician or other health professional to whom that authority is officially granted by the health plan. The requirement for referral is often called "gatekeeping," and the individual responsible for the authorization the "gatekeeper." In situations in which gatekeeping is required, self-referral by the patient, even with the recommendation of a physician not authorized by the health plan as a gatekeeper, will not result in reimbursement. (See Chapter 6 for more information on gatekeeping.)

In managed situations in which self-referral by the patient alone or referral at the recommendation of the primary care physician not subject to gatekeeping arrangements is allowed, the psychiatric care is still subject to utilization review. Thus, both avenues of access lead to subsequent review.

PRIOR REVIEW

Prior review, also known as *prior authorization* or *precertification*, is the advance evaluation of whether medical services proposed for a specific patient are consistent with the criteria of the health plan for determination of medical necessity. Prior review may include evaluation of the site or level of service of care, the duration of care, and the need for a specific procedure or service. Not every aspect of prior review is relevant to every patient. Prior review is most frequently required for inpatient care. In emergency situations, when prior review is not possible, review is usually required within 24–48 hours to certify the necessity of treatment (1).

Although prior review is most frequently required for inpatient care, it is increasingly employed in outpatient care, where authorization may be required in advance of treatment or after the first few visits, as specified in the health plan. In many HMOs and employee assistance programs (EAPs), prior review may be performed on a face-to-face basis between the patient and the health care professional officially designated by the plan to assess and refer the patient for treatment. In most fee-for-service utilization management, prior review is usually done by telephone and is between the psychiatrist and the first-level clinical reviewer, generally a psychiatric nurse or social worker. Written prior review requests are also in use and are preferred by some providers for the greater clarity and the historic record they may afford. Typically, prior review authorizes the initial procedures and initial amount, duration, and scope of service required to perform sufficient evaluation and to create a treatment plan. Submission of an initial treatment plan is required to follow quickly, and additional requests for service will be subject to concurrent review. In situations in which a patient has already been in outpatient treatment and a prior review is sought for more intensive outpatient or inpatient care, a more fully developed diagnosis, evaluation, and treatment plan will be required for the prior review.

Intensity of prior review varies according to the policy of the health plan and the level of care requested. Authorization for inpatient care is subjected to greater scrutiny than outpatient care. In all cases, the request should be as precise and descriptive as possible. Table 3–1 provides a general checklist of information requirements for prior review. Gathering as much of this information as possible and that is relevant to the patient in advance of the request will help to avoid frustrating and potentially harmful delays in authorization.

Again, prior review may authorize only sufficient service to initiate evaluation and assessment leading to the creation of a treatment plan, or it may authorize more substantial services for an established patient for whom initial assessment has already taken place. The amount of information required will vary accordingly. In both cases, prior authorization is followed by submission of a treatment plan, which will become the basis of subsequent review.

THE TREATMENT PLAN

The treatment plan, which is included in the medical record, distills the many assessments and evaluations into a coherent statement of the patient's diagnosis, deficits, and assets and establishes a series of treatment goals. It outlines the treatment program, including the specific treatment methods to be employed, the clinician(s) responsible for specific

Table 3–1. Checklist of information frequently requested for prior review

- Precipitants for seeking treatment at this time
- Diagnosis, or provisional diagnosis, using the multiaxial approach of DSM-III-R (2)
- Past history of present or other relevant conditions
- Goals of treatment
- Length of treatment anticipated to meet the goals
- Mechanisms that will be used to measure the patient's progress
- Level of treatment that will best enable the patient to reach those goals
- Services that will be used to achieve the treatment goals
- Initial discharge plan and how services will enable discharge
- Risk assessment including suicidal ideation, suicide attempts, or homicidal potential
- Medical complications
- Patient score on the Global Assessment of Functioning Scale (Axis V of DSM-III-R)
- Mental status examination and results of other physiological and psychiatric evaluations, if available

Source. Preferred Health Care: The PHC Manual: Clinical Protocols and Procedures. Wilton, CT, Preferred Health Care Ltd., 1990 (3).

segments of treatment, the time frames for reaching specific treatment objectives, and discharge criteria. Future review of the quality and appropriateness of the overall treatment process will begin with a review of the treatment plan. The treatment plan is submitted to the utilization management entity for approval. Only services consistent with the treatment plan will be authorized. Treatment will continue to be reviewed at intervals specified by the plan. The treatment plan thus becomes the basis for concurrent review. A checklist of information required for the treatment plan follows in Table 3–2.

Summary of a Treatment Plan: Administratively Successful

Symptoms on admission. Depressed, unable to function at job and home, unable to get out of bed, ruminative thoughts, overwhelming feelings of guilt, suicidal ideation, loss of appetite with weight loss of 30 pounds, sleeping 4–5 hours per night.

Current psychiatric diagnoses

Axis I.	Major depression, recurrent, with mood-congruent psychotic features
Axis II.	Avoidant personality
Axis III.	Weight loss, questionable etiology

Table 3–2.   Checklist of information frequently required for the treatment plan

---

- Presenting symptoms
- Diagnosis, using the multiaxial approach in DSM-III-R
- Goals of treatment
- Current treatment program including psychotherapy; medication management, if applicable; and assignment of responsibilities of the treatment team
- Response to treatment and summary of progress
- Necessity for continued treatment
- Plans for continued treatment
- Justification for level of care
- Discharge goals and criteria for discharge
- Estimated duration of treatment

Current treatment program.   Patient has been on the inpatient service for 1 week. She is being seen by me daily for psychotherapy and medical management of her depression. She is on imipramine 200 mg/day. Physical assessment is under way and thus far shows no organic etiology for her weight loss. She continues on a special nursing observation because of suicidal ideation. Social worker is seeing the family weekly in counseling.

Response to treatment.   Patient has begun to appear a bit more animated. She has begun to take some interest in her appearance. She spends less time lying in bed and has begun to talk with other patients. She is now sleeping up to 6 hours a night, though she still arises early. Her appetite remains poor. Patient has lost 2 pounds during the week.

Necessity for continued hospital treatment.   Despite minimal improvement, the patient remains profoundly depressed as demonstrated by her continued suicidal ruminations, psychomotor retardation, continued poor appetite, and minimal level of socialization and activity. Treatment and observation on an inpatient unit are required to monitor risk of suicide, to evaluate her response to treatment, and to initiate other treatments should the current regimen not be effective.

Plans for treatment.   Continued treatment with imipramine and assessment of response to a reasonable therapeutic trial. Possible change to other antidepressant medication or addition of lithium carbonate to therapeutic regimen if her clinical response is not satisfactory. Completion of physical assessment to rule out significant physical factors in weight loss. Continued treatment with psychotherapy to address interpersonal issues and social casework to address significant family issues that may have acted as precipitants to this episode.

Estimated length of stay.   Two weeks on the inpatient service. Patient will need ongoing psychiatric treatment and assessment on an ambulatory basis after discharge.

Summary of a Treatment Plan: Administratively Unsuccessful

Symptoms on admission.   Depressed and hopeless, no pleasure from activities, suicidal.

Current psychiatric diagnoses

Depression

Current treatment program. Patient has been on the inpatient service for 1 week. She is seeing me daily for psychotherapy and medication. She is attending classes in pottery and photography as part of a program of activity therapy.

Response to treatment. Patient seems better. She participates actively in psychotherapy, discussing at length her feelings of guilt over a past extramarital affair. She appears to be establishing a positive therapeutic relationship with me.

Necessity for continued hospital treatment. Despite some minimal improvement, the patient remains profoundly depressed. She needs more time to develop a solid therapeutic relationship, to work on her lifelong feelings of inadequacy, and to be away from the stressors at home.

Plans for treatment. Continued inpatient care and treatment with medication and psychotherapy.

Estimated length of stay. Impossible to tell at this early point in her treatment. She will be able to leave the hospital when she is no longer depressed.

CONCURRENT REVIEW

Concurrent review assesses the clinical justification of the initial authorization, the appropriateness of the treatment plan, the procedural consistency of services rendered with the measurable goals of treatment, and progress toward discharge planning. One concurrent review of the treatment plan is made even if no additional request for service is filed. If additional service requests for a continued inpatient stay or additional outpatient treatment beyond the initial authorization are made, they will be subject to additional concurrent reviews at specified intervals. The psychiatrist will be asked for written modified treatment plans, progress notes, and treatment summaries. These are then discussed via telephone between the psychiatrist and the reviewer. If these support approval of extended service for the patient, the reviewer will arrange for subsequent reviews at specific intervals.

The provider will be asked to send a copy of the psychiatrist's or other primary therapist's progress notes, treatment summary, and other records that are necessary to complete the reviewer's understanding of the case. It is important to note the difference between process notes and progress notes. *Process notes* are more detailed and depict the actual dialogue between the psychiatrist and the patient. They contain the actual dynamics and observations. Process notes should not be shared. *Progress notes* are less-detailed summaries of the accomplishments of the patient toward reaching the therapeutic goals. It is the progress notes that should be shared with the review entity. The review specialist will evaluate these records prior to a telephone interview with the responsible physician.

The treatment summaries and plan revisions should be directed toward fulfilling the criteria for discharge readiness contained in the discharge plan. It should be clear that the treatment team is considering the discharge criteria as related to the patient's ability to continue treatment in the community, not as arbitrary points of progress in a particular hospital privilege system or treatment model. The treatment team should be aware of planning the hospitalization course in accordance with the limits of a patient's insurance benefits and financial constraints. It may be necessary for the review specialist to be aware of benefit limitations before approving an extended stay. The treatment staff should inquire about possible financial limitations as part of their work with the family.

Table 3–3 provides a checklist of information frequently required for concurrent review.

PROCESS OBSERVATIONS

Determination of medical necessity drives the process of utilization management. To be deemed "necessary," a service must be

1. Adequate and essential for the evaluation and/or treatment of a disease, condition, or illness, as defined by standard diagnostic nomenclatures (ICD-9 [4] or DSM-III-R)
2. Reasonably expected to improve an individual's condition or level of functioning
3. In keeping with national standards of psychiatric practice as defined by standard clinical references, valid empirical experience for efficacy, and national professional standards promulgated by medical associations and federal agencies utilizing professional consensus development and scientific data

Utilization management entities usually require all three elements of medical necessity to be present throughout the course of treatment. Many add the requirement that treatment be provided at the most cost-effective level of care.

The need for precise information and clear language for authorization of service based on medical necessity cannot be overestimated. Utilization

---

Table 3–3. Checklist of information frequently required for concurrent review

---

- Any changes in diagnosis, comorbidities, etc.
- Changes in patient status that reflect progress or regression
- Any medical or neurological illness or treatment
- Current mental status and behavioral functioning, with changes since last review
- Special treatments such as suicide precautions or seclusion or restraint
- Any adverse behavioral episodes, such as self-injury, assaultive behavior, etc.
- A review of progress toward completion of each goal in the treatment plan and projection of the time frame for meeting the remaining goals; this should be contained in regular revisions of the plan by a team meeting with patient participation
- Progress in meeting goals of the discharge plan and any new goals for the plan
- The course of psychotherapy as it relates to the treatment plan, including the number and duration of sessions per week
- Family involvement, including number and duration of family therapy sessions and educational activities since the last review; this should be related to goals in the treatment plan
- Inpatient care and patient participation and progress in group, milieu activity, and educational or vocational rehabilitation therapies as they relate to the treatment plan
- The current medication regimen and explanations of any changes since the last review; special attention should be given to issues such as regular use of prn medication, routine use of hypnotics, regular monitoring of blood levels when appropriate, need for continued medication for extrapyramidal side effects, and efforts to achieve an optimal dose of medication

---

reviewers match the clinical information provided by the psychiatrist against the criteria for service developed by the utilization management company. Some utilization management companies reveal their criteria to physicians; most do not. The psychiatrist should always request the criteria and become familiar with them if the criteria are shared. If the criteria of a specific company are not available, the psychiatrist may turn to other sources for guidelines. The following publications may prove useful in gaining a general (although not company specific) sense of medical necessity and levels of care criteria.

- DSM-III-R (Washington, DC, American Psychiatric Association, 1987) (See especially "target symptoms") (2)
- *Manual of Psychiatric Peer Review*, 3rd Edition (Washington, DC, American Psychiatric Association, 1985) (5)
- *Manual of Psychiatric Quality Assurance* (Washington, DC, American Psychiatric Association, 1992) (6)
- *Guidelines for Treatment Resources in Quality Assurance, Peer Review and Reimbursement* (Washington, DC, American Academy of Child and Adolescent Psychiatry, 1990) (7)
- *The PHC Manual: Clinical Protocols and Procedures* (Wilton, CT, Preferred Health Care Ltd., 1990) (3)
- Hospital departments of quality assurance and utilization review may also have the medical necessity criteria for HMOs and managed care networks with whom they contract and Medicare peer review organization (PRO) requirements. These departments may be very helpful in making criteria available.

Criteria should be used accurately to facilitate communication with the reviewing body and to ascertain conditions of reimbursement at the time of treatment planning.

If the provider disagrees with the medical necessity criteria of the utilization management entity, appeal and/or provision of care without third-party payment may be necessary. Appeals and problems with utilization management are discussed subsequently in this chapter in the section "Denials and Appeals."

DISCHARGE PLANNING

Discharge planning for inpatients begins at the time of prior review of precertification and the allocation of the initial length of stay. Goals for discharge and follow-up care should be present in the initial treatment plan. Progress toward these discharge goals forms the basis for concurrent review decisions.

For outpatients, the equivalent of discharge planning is termination of treatment. Similar to inpatient discharge planning, goals for termination of treatment and suggestions for longer-term follow-up care and monitoring should be present in the initial treatment plan. Progress toward these goals constitutes the basis of concurrent review.

Discharge planning or termination of outpatient care may involve arrangements for additional follow-up medical and nonmedical services. Case management, which may be operative at any point in the patient's care, may be of great assistance in discharge planning.

CASE MANAGEMENT

Case management is a focused utilization management strategy targeted to relatively few beneficiaries who generate or are likely to generate very large expenditures or who require a large number of providers or services, possibly including social as well as medical services. Sometimes termed "large case management," "high-cost case management," or "individual benefits management," case management involves the assessment of the patient's health care needs as well as personal circumstances to determine whether extra assistance in planning, arranging, and coordinating a specialized treatment plan will permit appropriate and less costly care (1).

If the individual's health plan does not cover some elements of the treatment plan, individual exceptions to these coverage limitations may be approved through case management. Unlike utilization review, case management is voluntary and may permit coverage not specified in the benefit plan. For example, stays in residential facilities or partial hospital programs may be authorized to enable a patient to move from a more costly and restrictive setting to a cost-effective, less-restrictive alternative. Case management may be used at any point in the treatment plan.

RETROSPECTIVE REVIEW

Retrospective review is the final evaluation of utilization, designed to ensure consistency of the physician's treatment plan, progress reports, and the medical records. If there is inconsistency, denial of claims after services are rendered may occur. Prior and concurrent review have minimized the occurrence of much retrospective denial. Retrospective review usually takes the form of a medical record audit performed on-site for a random sample of patients. The results are primarily used for analyzing patterns of practitioner or institutional care for use in provider education, profiling, and selective contracting arrangements (1).

DENIALS AND APPEALS

Inherent in the process of authorization and case-by-case decision making is the prospect of denial of authorization for coverage and reimbursement of treatment.

Psychiatrists contracting with a managed care organization should carefully investigate the contract they sign for the articulation of the appeals process. When subject to review by outside utilization review organizations, one should request the appeals process in writing. There are two types of appeals: administrative and clinical.

Administrative Appeals

Unlike the better-known clinical appeal, in which the provider and reviewer disagree regarding medical necessity, administrative appeal addresses denial of coverage resulting from failure to comply with contract or procedural guidelines stipulated by the utilization management company. It is essential to discern the nature of the denial in order to appeal on appropriate grounds. Reasons for administrative denial may include

- Failure to obtain prior authorization at all, or within time constraints for emergency admissions
- Failure to furnish necessary clinical information
- Failure to comply with specified time frames
- Inappropriate referral to an out-of-network provider, if applicable
- Contractual exclusions of coverage
- Exhaustion of the benefit

Administrative appeal may be successful if unusual circumstances prevented compliance with administrative guidelines. Such mitigating circumstances may include inability of the patient to communicate insurance information while in need of imminent treatment. Denials resulting from exhaustion of the benefit may be addressed by requesting extension of benefits through case management and individual or flexible benefits management. (See the section "Case Management" in this chapter and Chapter 4, "Frequently Encountered Problems and Their Solutions" for more information.) Contractual exclusions of coverage are negotiated among the employer, the insurer, and the utilization management entity. There is little chance of appealing denial based on contractual exclusion. However, the patient may wish to discuss contractual exclusions with the employer for future redress.

Clinical Appeals

In clinical appeals, the provider seeks to reverse the decision of the review organization to deny certification of a service, procedure, admission, or extension of stay based on the failure of the request to meet the reviewer's criteria for medical necessity or level of care. Denial may occur at any point in the review process. Steps to avert denial have already been presented. If denial occurs, the following steps should be taken.

- Request written notification of the principal reason(s) for the determination and the way to initiate an appeal, including names and addresses of the appeal reviewers. Insist on a review by a psychiatrist who is board eligible, with subspecialty training as appropriate, who has experience with the treatment under consideration. (The initial discussion may begin via telephone in the course of a telephone review, but the information should still be requested in writing.)
- Review prior authorization or requests for extension of treatment for completeness, precision, and documentation; adjust as necessary.
- Study the reviewers' stated reason for denial.
- Address in the written appeal and subsequent telephone conversations the reasons for denial; supply additional clinical documentation or explanation of the treatment plan and reasons for your choice of treatment modalities and place of service; ask the reviewer for the utilization management entity's criteria; address these as appropriate.
- Exhaust all levels of appeal within the utilization management entity.
- If necessary, request referral to an external agency or specialist retained by the review organization for independent assessment; ascertain possible cost-sharing obligations for external review.
- Contact the American Psychiatric Association (APA) Managed Care Information Line (1-800-343-4671) for advice.
- In emergency situations, request an "expedited appeal." If precertification for urgent care is denied or denial occurs during an ongoing service, the attending psychiatrist should request the opportunity to appeal the denial over the telephone on an expedited basis. Make clear to the reviewer that you are requesting an expedited appeal and that you must speak to the consulting psychiatrist immediately. (You will still need to complete the paperwork.)
- Expedited appeals that are not granted should be resubmitted through the standard appeals process.
- Observe all time requirements for the appeals process.

It is the ethical obligation of the treating physician to provide medically necessary care, stabilization, and transfer or arrangements for additional care. Denial of authorization for reimbursement by a payer or review organization does not release a provider from the ethical obligation to provide necessary care during or after the denial or appeals process. In addition, although some recent legal decisions have included the payer or review organization in liability for negative outcomes resulting from failure to reimburse for care, the provider has not been exempted from liability. It is the physicians' ethical and legal responsibility to provide or arrange for necessary care.

If the complete appeals process fails

- Continue to provide or arrange for necessary care.
- Pursue the grievance at the policy level with
  - The APA Managed Care Information Line (1-800-343-4671)
  - The district branch liaison to the APA Managed Care Network
  - The corporate headquarters of the utilization management company
  - The state insurance commission
- The patient may wish to discuss grievances with his or her employer (about management of the insurance plan).

SUMMARY OBSERVATIONS

Communication, dialogue, and documentation are the keys to successful navigation of the review process. It is impossible to overestimate the importance of communication, including diagnostic specificity, precise descriptions of patient characteristics, clarity of treatment goals and treatment progress, the consistency between treatment goals and discharge planning, and the necessity for open, good-faith dialogue between the psychiatrist and the reviewer.

CHAPTER 4

FREQUENTLY ENCOUNTERED
PROBLEMS AND THEIR SOLUTIONS

CLINICAL PROBLEMS

Problem. *You provide the appropriate information to the reviewer, which in your opinion meets medical necessity criteria for a certain level of care. The reviewer thanks you for your information but then refuses to authorize payment for care.*

Solution. Ask the reviewer for the utilization management entity's definition of medical necessity, standard of care, and criteria for the problem specified. If this is not satisfactory, demand to speak to the reviewer's supervisor. If the reviewer is not a psychiatrist, insist on that level of review. The reviewing psychiatrist should be experienced in the type of treatment being reviewed.

Problem. *If, after speaking to the reviewing psychiatrist, you are still not satisfied, where can you go?*

Solution. Ask the managed care director about the appeals mechanism. Exhaust all appeals. If you are still not satisfied, consider contacting your state insurance commissioner (see Appendix 3) or, with your patient's permission, the benefits representative and/or employee assistance program (EAP) of the company being managed.

Problem. *Your hospitalized psychotic patient refuses any medication and the reviewing psychiatrist tells you that if the patient is refusing care, payment will not be authorized.*

Solution. In any cases in which you feel the reviewing psychiatrist is interfering with your practice of medicine and/or specifically instructing you on which medication to prescribe, you may want to go out of the system entirely for redress. This may mean contacting the corporate medical director of the managed care company (see Appendix 1) to file a complaint or the American Psychiatric Association (APA) Managed Care Information Line (1-800-343-4671). In this example, antipsychotic medication is the treatment of choice. However, we would also agree that without court intervention, patients cannot be forced to take medication. While waiting for the court ruling, the patient will continue to need 24-hour medical supervision, and it is not possible to discharge the patient.

Problem. *You are providing outpatient care for a patient, and the crisis symptoms have subsided. You now would like to work on long-term character-changing issues, but the managed care reviewer tells you that this is medically unnecessary.*

Solution. You must understand your contract before you sign it. If the emphasis is on only short-term crisis intervention, you may have no recourse. If you appeal, understand that you may be requested to cite medical references. You may wish to continue treatment with your patient outside of the insurance benefit. In this case, the contract will have to be between you and your patient for payment of care.

OPERATIONAL PROBLEMS

Problem. *The patient has used all of the benefits but still needs care (this applies to inpatient and outpatient care).*

Solution. Depending on the insurance benefit design, you may be able to negotiate continued care. This may occur if you can demonstrate that continued treatment will improve the patient's functioning and prevent hospitalization. It is less likely to work if the patient is receiving care for a chronic condition.

Problem. *The patient is in treatment and has been approved at the appropriate level of care by the managed care company, and continuation of treatment is being questioned. An independent reviewer wants to come to the hospital and visit your patient.*

Solution. Depending on the benefit design of the contract, there may be a provision allowing the managed care reviewer to read the chart. In unusual circumstances, an independent review may be allowed. This usually occurs only in patients hospitalized over a long period, who have failed in a number of different treatment protocols. Before such a review takes place, there should be consensus between the patient's physician, the treatment center, and the reviewer on the setting, type of review, length of time for the review, and the relationship of this independent review and any further treatment. The outside reviewer should agree not to provide any treatment, prescriptions, or recommendations to the patient. You should be able to observe this review.

Problem. *You are concerned about confidential information that you have given to the managed care company being leaked to the employer or other agents.*

Solution. It is a violation of medical ethics, federal laws, and many state statutes to provide certain information without written permission from the patient. You and your patient may pursue this through the managed care–corporate relationship or through other civil actions.

Problem. *You spend more than 30 seconds waiting for the managed care company to answer the telephone or when they do answer the telephone you find that an inordinate amount of your time is taken to make determinations concerning medical necessity issues.*

Solution. You may express dissatisfaction to the directors of the managed care program (see Appendix 1), their corporate clients, or the APA Managed Care Information Line (1-800-343-4671). The APA will compile these complaints. If there are a number of them, The Committee on Managed Care of the APA will make a formal complaint to the medical director of the specific managed care program.

Problem. *You are uncomfortable with the managed care reviewer. You have questions about his or her training, expertise, and competence. You feel that the interview was handled in an unprofessional fashion.*

Solution. You may express dissatisfaction through the directors of the managed care program, their corporate clients, or the APA Managed Care Information Line (1-800-343-4671). The APA will compile these complaints. If there are a number of them, The Committee on Managed Care of the APA will make a formal complaint to the medical director of the managed care program.

FINANCIAL PROBLEMS

Problem. *How do you charge the managed care company for your time?*

Solution. If you are in a preferred provider organization (PPO) in which you agree to participate in managed care as part of accepting their patients on a referral basis, you cannot charge for your time. If the patient is insured by a company that insists on utilization review and/or managed care, and you are not part of the PPO, you may wish to charge the patient or the insurer. This should be negotiated before the lengthy review process takes place. To date, very few practitioners bill or are paid for their telephone time.

Problem. *You are dissatisfied with funds paid to you by the carrier for provision of care.*

Solution. This is a complicated issue that has a number of variables. Often fees are negotiated for large groups, and, if you agree to accept this negotiated fee, it is not alterable during the fixed period that the program is in place. When the program is in review for renewal of the contract, this is a good time to renegotiate the fees. If you are a nonparticipating provider who is caring for a managed care patient, you should be able to bill the patient the amount not covered by the patient's insurance. This should be discussed with your patient before and during provision of the service.

Problem. *Your hospital agrees to a contract with the managed care company, including a flat daily rate that includes your fees.*

Solution. You may refuse to care for these patients, negotiate with your hospital what percentage of a daily fee will be funded to you, or take a salaried job at the hospital. If you bill the patient, your bill will be rejected.

CHAPTER 5

CONFIDENTIALITY

Because of increasing demands to release information to third parties, the information in a medical record should be limited to that which is necessary to meet the requirements of law and to maintain a documented data base appropriate for continued treatment. Extraneous and irrelevant materials should be kept to a minimum, as should material that is sensitive or potentially damaging to the patient or other persons.

The psychiatrist may keep informal personal work notes on a given case, independent of the official medical record. These should be kept physically separate from the medical record and should not be used as a substitute for it. Psychiatrists can record their impressions and speculations in these work notes, as well as verbatim and process notations, other sensitive information, and information from third parties. Psychiatrists should be aware, however, that such personal notes are protected from disclosure only in a limited number of jurisdictions.

PATIENT ACCESS TO RECORDS

In the current atmosphere of increased participation by patients in their own care, requests are often made that patients be given their own records or be permitted access to them. Actual medical records made and maintained by psychiatrists belong to them or to the clinics or hospitals in which they work, and there is no obligation to relinquish them to patients. In many jurisdictions, however, the patient has the right to inspect and/or have a copy of the medical record on request. Some states limit this access and permit the psychiatrist to withhold from the patient information that would have a negative impact on his or her health or well-being, although the record must be released to other physicians of the patient's choosing.

Psychiatrists should become familiar with the laws governing patient access to records in the jurisdictions in which they practice.

RELEASE OF RECORDS TO A THIRD PARTY

Psychiatrists and other physicians are constantly asked by a variety of third parties to release information about their patients. The majority of these release requests are from insurance carriers, but they may also be from other health care providers, from administrative bodies, and from various components of the legal system. Generally, such a request is accompanied by a written authorization signed by the patient. Many states have statutes that address the form and duration of consent, the type of information that may be released, and restrictions governing disclosure. Psychiatrists should thus familiarize themselves with any special provisions that apply in the jurisdictions in which they practice.

No information about patients should be released to parties not directly involved in their care without their explicit, written permission unless such releases are required by law or by court order. The patient's consent to the release of information from his or her medical record should be informed and given freely, without threat or coercion. In practice, however, this is often not the case. To receive insurance benefits to which they are otherwise entitled, for example, patients are frequently requested to sign open-ended blanket releases without restriction on the type of information to be released. For their consent to be informed, patients should appreciate the nature and content of the information to be released, the purposes for which it will be used, the manner in which it will be protected, and the extent to which any of the information may be redisclosed to other parties. Logically, it is not possible to give a fully informed authorization before the care itself has been rendered and the patient has had an opportunity to review the information involved. Authorizations that accompany requests for release of information, however, frequently predate much of the information requested.

In the absence of clear legal guidelines on how to proceed when the authorization for the release of information is questionable, the psychiatrist should take care to protect the patient's interests. If he or she has any questions about whether the patient understood the nature and extent of the disclosure involved or is concerned about the release of sensitive or harmful material, the psychiatrist should contact the patient and discuss these matters before releasing information. As always, the psychiatrist should take care to limit the information disclosed to that which is relevant to the particular purpose of the request.

Psychiatrists may occasionally receive requests for information about patients over the telephone or through other informal channels. Except in matters of medical emergency, no release of information should be made without the patient's specific approval and no information should be given or sent to anyone unless the psychiatrist has reasonable certainty of that individual's identity. A psychiatrist should not acknowledge that an individual is or was under his or her care without the patient's specific approval.

Sharing Records With Consulting Health Care Professionals and Agencies

Generally, the sharing of clinical information with a consultant directly involved in the care of a given patient does not require specific authorization, provided that the patient has approved of the consultation. Similarly, a letter of referral to another health care professional or a letter in reply to such a referral does not need specific authorization if the patient has approved the referral. Care must always be taken to limit materials sent through the mail and to indicate clearly that the material is "personal and confidential" for the addressee. Where there is any doubt about the appropriateness of sharing clinical information about a patient with another professional, a release from the patient should be obtained.

Many practitioners and psychiatric clinics have formal joint service and consultative arrangements with other health care providers that involve conjoint care of certain patients. Whenever clinical information is shared between such practitioners and agencies, written agreements should be developed that specify the amount and type of material that may be transmitted between them in providing collaborative care. Patients should be notified of the arrangements and have the option of having their records not shared in this manner, even if this deters optimum care.

Redisclosure of Records

Psychiatrists may possess copies of patients' medical records that have been obtained from other health care providers. Patients' authorizations for psychiatrists to release information to other parties do not cover the release of these records unless they are specifically included in the release and their rerelease is not otherwise prohibited.

The laws about redisclosure of medical information that has been sent to insurance companies, government agencies, and others not involved in providing health care are much less clear. In many instances, these bodies are not legally prohibited from releasing medical information to other parties. The ever-present possibility of such redisclosure should caution psychiatrists to be extremely prudent about the information released to these organizations and agencies. Nonmedical agencies and organizations are not bound by the same ethical standards as health professionals regarding the confidentiality of medical records that come into their possession. Although most take reasonable precautions to protect such data, access to these data is not formally regulated and redisclosure to other parties may occur with relative ease.

TELEPHONE REVIEW[*]

The use of telephone interviews for the conduct of utilization review has grown rapidly during the 1980s and into the 1990s and has created new concerns about confidentiality. The most immediate concern is the identity of the person calling the treating physician and that person's right to gain access to clinical information. The treating psychiatrist can take several steps to confirm the identity of the caller, such as

- Questioning the caller for information that would only be available to a review organization (e.g., the patient's policy number or group insurance identification number)
- Returning the call to the review organization's published telephone number
- Calling the insurance company to confirm the legitimacy of the review organization

The next concern is the patient's informed consent to this type of review. Informed legal opinion holds that the blanket consent form usually signed by the patient when obtaining health insurance is sufficient to authorize the psychiatrist's communication with the insurance company and its review organization. However, this blanket consent form may not actually constitute informed consent. The psychiatrist should discuss the nature of the telephone review process with the patient and obtain signed consent to speak with the review organization. The patient should understand that the telephone interview may require disclosure of detailed clinical information. The patient may wish to limit disclosure of certain

---

[*]Reprinted with permission from Deutschman DA: Telephone review, in *Manual of Psychiatric Quality Assurance.* Washington, DC, American Psychiatric Association, 1992, p. 49. Copyright 1992 American Psychiatric Association.

information, but the patient must also be aware that failure to obtain approval may have an adverse economic impact.

Some psychiatrists are concerned that the telephone review process forces disclosure of much more information than past methods utilizing claim forms or written peer review reports. They believe that this disclosure may interfere with the process of intensive psychotherapy. This concern about disclosure of information to an insurance company has led some patients to avoid treatment or to decide not to file insurance claims. A patient's worry may be alleviated significantly if the psychiatrist and patient agree beforehand on the limits they will place on the issues or the personal information that the psychiatrist will be able to disclose.

Similarly, patients of self-insured employers that have engaged a utilization review company to manage care are concerned that the clinical information obtained by a reviewer may be accessible to the employer. This is an issue in any form of review, but concern may be heightened due to the greater intensity and frequency possible with telephonic review. The patient has the responsibility to evaluate this risk and to determine the amount of information to be released.

CONTRACTING

A physician or provider contract is a legal agreement that imposes binding responsibilities for both parties (the provider and the managed care organization) signing the document. A contract with a managed care firm usually includes reimbursement procedures (i.e., fee-for-service, fee schedules, or capitation), utilization review activities, referral patterns, and liability.

It is always advisable to have an attorney examine a provider contract with any business entity before signing. It is recommended to use an attorney who is familiar with health care contracts and knowledgeable about the practices and philosophies of managed care. American Psychiatric Association (APA) members can also contact the APA legal counsel. Members may participate in an APA legal plan, or they can contact counsel directly. Legal advice to individuals is provided at the physician's own expense.

The contracts should include the definitions and explanations of the terms of the agreement. In this chapter, issues concerning provider contracting are presented in five major categories: legal, financial, organizational, operational, and utilization review.

LEGAL CONSIDERATIONS

Term of Contract

The term of a provider contract is usually 1 year, with annual renewals available. Common language describing the term of the contract is "the term of this Agreement shall be for a period of one (1) year and shall therefore be extended for successive periods of twelve (12) months, unless terminated by either party."

Significant portions of this chapter are adapted from the *Marketing Manual for District Branches* of the American Psychiatric Association.

Termination

Most contracts can be terminated by either party with 60 days' notice; some also provide for a shorter termination period in the event of a breach of contract by one of the parties. Some plans may require a physician to continue to treat patients after termination of the contract, although the time period may not be long. In this case, the physician's ability to terminate the contract is tied to the patient contract. A provider agreement should be written so that either party can terminate the contract.

Another issue regarding termination should be mentioned. If a managed care organization should fail financially, the physician may still be legally required to continue to provide care to a patient who is a subscriber of the plan.

Professional Liability

Professional liability is the legal and financial obligation of a physician to compensate a patient for injury that results from the physician's treatment or failure to provide treatment. All health maintenance organization (HMO) contracts require physicians to carry independent malpractice insurance. Typically, the contract requires the physician to maintain liability insurance equal to or greater than that required by 1) the state, 2) the hospital at which the physician has admitting privileges, 3) the board of directors of the plan, or 4) community standards.

"Hold Harmless" Clauses

The "hold harmless" clause shifts responsibilities for any contractual liability to the physician; the physician agrees to hold the managed care organization "harmless" for any liability arising from the contract. Physicians' professional liability insurance coverage usually excludes any liability assumed under contract or agreement.

Provider contracts stipulate that the physician will be subject to the utilization review procedures of the managed care firm. However, the managed care firm's refusal to authorize treatment will not excuse the physician who fails to provide medically necessary care. The firm may still carry independent responsibility, but the physician is not exempt from liability by accepting the decision of the managed care firm.

Peer Review Liability

Provider contracts often require physicians to participate in peer review. Physicians involved in peer review activities such as hospital medical staffs or medical society committees are usually granted legal protections from liability by their state. However, peer review done for cost-containment reasons rather than to ensure the quality of medical care may not have this immunity. Physicians should determine if a contract requires peer review activity and if that is covered by their liability insurance.

Compliance With the Federal Trade Commission

The federal government is increasingly investigating allegations of antitrust in provider contracts. Physicians should have an attorney review all contracts to determine that signing such a contract will not open the physician to antitrust legislation. The Federal Trade Commission has taken particular interest in enforcing antitrust laws concerning provider boycotts of managed care plans. Although an independent practice association (IPA) can present information about a managed care firm to its members, each physician must decide to contract or not to contract individually.

Another issue that the government has raised is provider reimbursement. To avoid any suspicion of price-fixing, it is advisable not to discuss fees with other physicians. In addition, providers should not interfere with other provider's rights to practice or earn a living.

Exclusivity

An exclusivity clause in a provider contract requires that one or both of the parties agree to contract only with each other—and no other competitors. Some managed care plans have asked for exclusive arrangements with certain physician groups. This issue is becoming less common as providers contract with multiple organizations.

FINANCIAL CONSIDERATIONS

Provider Reimbursement

Managed care firms have used a variety of methods to reimburse physicians for their services. The provider contract should identify the method of reimbursement and provide more detailed information (e.g., a schedule of fees), if appropriate. The most common physician reimbursement mechanisms are

- Fixed-fee schedule
- Discounted fee-for-service
- Capitation

In a fixed-fee schedule, all physicians receive the same payment for the same procedures, based on either an average of fees in the area or a relative value scale. A discounted fee-for-service arrangement simply indicates that physicians are asked to discount a certain percentage (usually 10%–20%) off their regular fees. In a contract that specifies reimbursement by capitation, physicians are paid a certain amount per number of enrollees in the plan.

Many provider contracts include a "withhold" on physician reimbursement. A withhold requires a percentage (e.g., 10%) of the physician's fees to be reserved until the end of the contract. That amount could also be placed at risk; the physician receives the reserved payment only if the business is profitable. In this type of contract, if the firm lost money, the provider would not receive the withheld fees.

Billing Procedures

In provider contracts, a physician must agree to accept the insurer's fee for services rendered. If a physician's normal charge exceeds the fee, the physician cannot bill the patient for the remainder, unless a copayment of coinsurance is so documented in the subscriber/enrollee's contract. If a plan includes copayments, the physician must bill the insurer for the agreed-on fee and bill the patient for the copayment. (In an HMO, a copayment may be $10–$20 per visit or treatment; coinsurance may be 20% of a visit or treatment.)

It is also important to be aware of the managed care organization's coding system. Most insurers require use of the CPT-4 procedure codes and may require use of the ICD-9 (4) diagnostic coding system in lieu of DSM-III-R (2).

Payment Schedule

Preferred provider organizations (PPOs) and HMOs often claim to provide much quicker payment of fees (e.g., 30 days) than indemnity plans, but many contracts do not specify the payment schedule.

ORGANIZATIONAL CONSIDERATIONS

Gatekeeper

Most managed care plans utilize the concept of a "gatekeeper" for referral to a specialist. The patient must be referred to a specialist by a primary care provider who is participating in the plan, or the plan might not pay for the medical service. A patient can seek a physician without going through the gatekeeper, but risks not being reimbursed by the plan. Physicians should also be aware that managed care firms often use a different name for a gatekeeper, for example, "patient care manager." The gatekeeper may be the patient's own primary care provider or, in some cases, a mental health provider specifically designated by the health plan. In the latter case, the patient must receive authorization for psychiatric treatment from a gatekeeper other than the primary care physician. It is essential to familiarize oneself with the gatekeeping process in all of the plans with which one participates.

Current Hospital and Physician Contracts

Psychiatrists who are contemplating signing with a managed care organization should ask for a list of providers (hospitals and physicians) who have currently contracted with the firm. In this way, a physician can determine if the contract hospitals are the same facilities that the physician uses.

Referral Resources

Many managed care firms limit referrals to "contract" providers (physicians who are participating in the plan). Referring to noncontracting physicians, or admitting to noncontracting hospitals, may result in an unreimbursed expense to the patient. In cases in which the carrier has failed to arrange for adequate resources, the physician will have to carefully document the problem and may need to assist the patient in forcing the carrier to accept responsibility.

OPERATIONAL CONSIDERATIONS

State Certification

Every state has passed laws or approved regulations to certify and/or regulate HMOs. Many states have also developed regulations on PPOs and other managed care organizations. The plans should meet all necessary requirements and be considered in good standing with the state.

Federal Qualification

Federal qualification for HMOs may not be as important now as in the past, because the states have improved their certification process. Many plans now opt for state certification over federal qualification due to fewer restrictions with state certification, often allowing more competitive rates. Whereas employers and unions previously required federal qualification, most now accept state certification.

Current Number of Enrollees

The current number of enrollees can serve as a predictor of the potential number of patients. Also, depending on the age of the plan, the number of enrollees indicates the favorability of the plan by health care purchasers and possibly its financial situation.

Service Area

Managed care plans, such as HMOs and PPOs, usually determine their service area by zip codes. Obviously, the plan's service area needs to overlap the physician's service area to provide a sufficient number of potential patients.

Current Major Employer/Employee Groups

Most managed care organizations will state which major employers have contracted with the firm for health care services. This can give the physician an indication of 1) the acceptance of the plan by the major purchasers of health care, 2) the number of potential patients, and 3) whether the signed enrollees are current patients (e.g., if the physician sees a significant number of employees from a specific large firm).

UTILIZATION REVIEW CONSIDERATIONS

The contract should contain very specific language as to the physician's obligations to the plan's utilization review program. The information should be contained in the body of the contract, not only in an addendum to the contract. The provider contractor should also identify the lines of responsibility for the plan's utilization review program and should indicate the professional level of the review coordinators: psychiatrist, social worker, or nurse. An expanded discussion of the utilization review process is found in Chapter 3.

REFERENCES

1. Institute of Medicine: Controlling Costs and Changing Patient Care: The Role of Utilization Management. Washington, DC, National Academy Press, 1989
2. American Psychiatric Association: Diagnostic and Statistical Manual of Mental Disorders, 3rd Edition, Revised. Washington, DC, American Psychiatric Association, 1987
3. Preferred Health Care: The PHC Manual: Clinical Protocols and Procedures. Wilton, CT, Preferred Health Care Ltd., 1990
4. International Classification of Diseases, 9th Revision. Geneva, World Health Organization, 1978
5. American Psychiatric Association: Manual of Psychiatric Peer Review, 3rd Edition. Washington, DC, American Psychiatric Association, 1985
6. American Psychiatric Association: Manual of Psychiatric Quality Assurance. Washington, DC, American Psychiatric Association, 1992
7. American Academy of Child and Adolescent Psychiatry: Guidelines for Treatment Resources in Quality Assurance, Peer Review and Reimbursement. Washington, DC, American Academy of Child and Adolescent Psychiatry, 1990

APPENDIXES

The following appendixes are included as further resources for the psychiatrist in working with managed care. Appendixes 1, 2, and 3 contain the names and addresses of chief executive officers or medical directors of major managed care and utilization review companies, major health insurance companies, and state insurance commissioners. These are offered to facilitate communication with these entities. Appendix 4 is a selected bibliography of publications in quality assurance, utilization review, and managed care, offered as an educational resource.

Chief Executive Officers
of Major Managed Care and
Utilization Review Companies

Arizona

Cori Hamilton
Action Health Care, Inc.
301 E. Bethany Road
Suite C278
Phoenix, AZ 85012

California

Robert Glaza
American Benefit Plan
  Administrators, Inc.
2999 W. Sixth Street
Los Angeles, CA 90020

Albert Waxman
American Biodyne Inc.
400 Oyster Point Boulevard
Suite 306
South San Francisco, CA 94080

Julie Bigelow
August International Corp.
One City Boulevard West
Suite 1000
Orange, CA 92668

Anita Vitale-Geist
Beech Street, Inc.
2 Ada
Irvine, CA 92718

Thomas Paton
Blue Shield of California
2 North Point Plaza
San Francisco, CA 94133

Dr. E. Scott Rosenblum
President
Business Health Services, Inc.
7311 Greenhaven Drive
Sacramento, CA 95831

Dr. Edward Zalta
Capp Care, Inc.
17390 Brookhurst
Suite 280
Fountain Valley, CA 92708

Martha Silvany
Care Resources, Inc.
20520 Nordhoff
Chatsworth, CA 91311

Larry Gallant
President
Coast Medical Review, Inc.
12235 Beach Boulevard
Suite 9
Stanton, CA 90680

Larry Goelman
Cost Care, Inc.
17011 Beach Boulevard
Huntington Beach, CA 92647

Elaine Hislop
Executive Director
Health Care Evaluation, Inc.
1212 W. Robinhood Drive
Suite 3-D
Stockton, CA 95207

Dr. Donald K. Kelly
Health International, Inc.
1840 Century Park E.
Suite 670
Los Angeles, CA 90067

Ellie Brokaw
HealthWatch Medical Review
  System
850 Town & Country Road
Orange, CA 92702

Ron Holman, Ph.D.
President
The Holman Group
6900 Owensmouth Avenue
Canoga Park, CA 91303

Raymond E. Hughes
Chairman
Managed Care Administrators
12651 High Bluee Drive
Suite 203
San Diego, CA 92130

Dr. Arnold Milstein
President
National Medical Audit
3 Embarcadero Center
Suite 1250
San Francisco, CA 94111

Vicki Merrill
Pacific Review Services
5995 Plaza Drive
Cypress, CA 90630-0848

Dr. Alvin Saidiner
PCC/Drug Data Systems, Inc.
828 Hollywood Way
Burbank, CA 91505

Suzanne Moore
President
SCM Associates, Inc.
9315 Vista Bonita
Cypress, CA 90630

Daniel Wilner, Ph.D.
University Healthcare
  Marketing, Inc.
1316 Theyer Avenue
P.O. Box 24-1590
Los Angeles, CA 90024

Stuart Grochowski
U.S. Administrators, Inc.
3540 Wilshire Boulevard
Los Angeles, CA 90010

Donald P. Balzano
Western Medical Review
  (Care Resource, Inc.)
23840 Hawthorne Boulevard
Torrance, CA 90505

COLORADO

Dr. Tom Barrett
Executive Director
Bethesda Provider Organization
5200 DTC Parkway
Suite 510
Englewood, CO 80111

Iva Conner
Great-West Life Assurance Co./
  Health Review Service
8505 E. Orchard Road
Englewood, CO 80111

CONNECTICUT

Paul Frankel, M.D.
Corporate Health Strategies
275 Post Road W.
Westport, CT 06880

Dr. Jay Reibel
Chairman
Preferred Health Care Ltd.
15 River Road
Wilton, CT 06897

Marcia Petrillo
Quality Care Review, Inc.
100 Roscommon Drive
Middletown, CT 06457

Robert E. Patricelli
President
Value Health Inc.
22 Waterville Road
Avon, CT 06001

DISTRICT OF COLUMBIA

E. Seton Shields
President
Health Management Strategies
  International, Inc.
1301 Pennsylvania Avenue, N.W.
Suite 800
Washington, DC 20004

Daniel O'Sullivan
President
Zenith Administrators
111 Massachusetts Avenue, N.W.
Washington, DC 20001

FLORIDA

Dennis Huffman
ConServCo
3903 Northdale Boulevard
Suite 200
Tampa, FL 33624

Leonard Russo
Chief Executive Officer
Cost Containment Management
5401 W. Kennedy Boulevard
Suite 271
Tampa, FL 33609

Marlene Mahle
Executive Director
Healthlink Review Corp.
6278 N. Federal Highway
Suite 155
Fort Lauderdale, FL 33308

John Sforza
Medical Foundation Services, Inc.
3625 N.W. 82nd Avenue
Suite 211
Miami, FL 33168

Dr. Julio Avello
President
Mental Health Management
7950 N.W. 53rd Street
Suite 204
Miami, FL 33166

Lois Hansen
National Health Network, Inc.
933 Lee Road
Suite 300
Orlando, FL 32810

GEORGIA

Jeff Aycock
Crawford & Co
P.O. Box 5047
Atlanta, GA 30302

Dr. Berk Lynch
Crawford Health Management
7 East Congress Street
Suite 400
P.O. Box 9507
Savannah, GA 31412

S. Walker McCune
Executive Vice-President
UMP
1718 Peachtree Street, N.W.
Suite 552
Atlanta, GA 30309

ILLINOIS

Gloria Siegel
Associated Agencies, Inc.
651 W. Washington Boulevard
Chicago, IL 60606

Dr. Ronald Kirschner
Association for Organization
  & Human Development
1701 Lake Avenue
Glenview, IL 60025

F. Jerome Cogwillard
CareAmerica, Inc.
301 E. Main Street
Suite 114
Barrington, IL 60010

Louis R. Morgan
DataMed, Inc.
650 W. Dandee Road
Northbrook, IL 60062

Stephanie Kramer
Efficient Health Systems, Inc.
5215 Old Orchard Road
Suite 360
Skokie, IL 60077

Dr. Robert Becker
HealthCare Compare Corp.
3200 Highland Avenue
Downers Grove, IL 60515

Richard Daly
The Health Data Institute—
  Management Care Division
900 N. State Parkway
Suite 325
Schaamburg, IL 60173

George C. Phillips, Jr.
President
HealthNetwork, Inc.
1420 Kensington Road
Suite 203
Oak Brook, IL 60521

Michael Kepple
Kepple & Company, Inc.
1811 W. Altorfer Drive
Peoria, IL 61615

Michael J. O'Connor
Medical Cost Management Corp.
122 S. Michigan Avenue
Suite 1200
Chicago, IL 60604

Jenifer Cline
Vice-President
Parkside Health Management
  Corp.
205 W. Touhy Avenue
Park Ridge, IL 60068

William Werner, M.D.
Republic-RSB Cos., Inc.
Park Street
Naperville, IL 60540

Robert M. Schrayer
President
RMSCO Management Services,
  Inc.
651 W. Washington Boulevard
Chicago, IL 60606

Jane Ballenger
Rush Contract Care
910 W. Van Buren Street
Chicago, IL 60607

INDIANA

Cynthia Dorell
Key Care Health Resources
5587 W. 73rd Street
Indianapolis, IN 46268

Barry J. Sullivan
President
Sagamore Health Network, Inc.
11555 N. Meridian Street
Suite 400
Carmel, IN 46032

IOWA

Rebecca Hemann
The Sunderbruch Corp.
3737 Woodland Avenue
Suite 622
West Des Moines, IA 50265

KANSAS

Gail Shafton
CarreFour Managed Health Care
7930 State Line Road
Suite 214
Prairie Village, KS 66208

KENTUCKY

James C. Rogers
President
Healthcare Review Corp.
9200 Shelbyville Road
Suite 215
Louisville, KY 40222

Wayne Smith
Humana Health Care Plans
500 W. Main Street
P.O. Box 1438
Louisville, KY 40201

Thomas Wannemuehler, L.C.S.W.
Wayne & Associates, Inc.
Suite 1166 Medical Arts Building
Louisville, KY 40217

LOUISIANA

Katherine Belchic
Associated Medical Review
  Services, Inc.
2821 Richland Avenue
Metairie, LA 70002

MAINE

Mary Orloski
Health Resources Ltd.
3 N.P.O. Box 246
Lancy Street
Pittsfield, ME 04967

MARYLAND

Anne Glenn
American International Health
  Care
7811 Montrose Road
Potomac, MD 20854

Paul Shaffeitt, M.D.
GreenSpring Mental Health
  Services
Park Side
Suite 700
10500 Little Patuxent Parkway
Columbia, MD 21044

Janice K. Albert
President
HealthCare Strategies, Inc.
9841 Broken Land Parkway
Suite 105
Columbia, MD 21046

Ronald E. Gots
National Medical Advisory
  Service
7910 Woodmont Avenue
#700
Bethesda, MD 20814

Joseph Lynaugh
Sanus Preferred Services
6611 Kenilworth Avenue
#300
Riverdale, MD 20737

William H. Slavin
Chief Executive Officer
United HealthCare, Inc.
2811 Lord Baltimore Drive
Baltimore, MD 21207

MASSACHUSETTS

Rick Kinyon
Assured Health Systems Inc.
20 Mall Road
Suite 130
Burlington, MA 01803

Donald D. Gilligan
President
Biotrak Marketing Group, Inc.
Building 600
1 Kendall Square
Cambridge, MA 02139

Arny Spielberg
HealthPro, Inc.
10 Mechanic Street
Worcester, MA 01608

Jerry Boyer
Managed Health Care
P.O. Box 11
Boston, MA 02117

Tera Younger
Executive Director
Massachusetts Peer Review
  Organization (MassPRO)
300 Bear Hill Road
P.O. Box 9007
Waltham, MA 02254

Russel Robbins
Peer Review Analysis, Inc.
380 Pleasant Street
Malden, MA 02148

MICHIGAN

Kathleen Etienne
President
Coordinated Rehabilitation
  Services, Inc.
4740 Marsh
Okemos, MI 48864

Jane Esenwein McCreary
Health Management Services, Inc.
5181 Cascade Road, S.E.
Grand Rapids, MI 49506

Robert J. Mackey
MedView/CompPRO
30057 Orchard Lake Road
Farmington Hills, MI 48018

MINNESOTA

Barbara Hayslip
HealthMarc, Inc.
5601 Smetna Drive
Suite 400
Minneapolis, MN 55343

Dr. Gary McIlroy
Health Risk Management, Inc.
8000 W. 78th Street
Suite 270
Minneapolis, MN 55343

John Bartlett, M.D.
MCC
1401 W. 76th Street
Suite 400
Minneapolis, MN 55423

Ronald G. Cameron
Medtrac, Inc.
2550 University Avenue
Suite 240N
St. Paul, MN 55114

Mary Young
United Behavioral Services, Inc.
3600 W. 80th Street
Suite 360
Minneapolis, MN 55431

MISSOURI

Patrick A. Thompson
Cost Management Technologies
4435 Main Street
Suite 810
Kansas City, MO 64111

NEBRASKA

Wesley Wilhelm, M.D.
Mutual of Omaha Insurance Co.
Mutual of Omaha Plaza
Omaha, NE 68175

NEVADA

Dr. Elias F. Ghanem
President
C.U.R.B. Associates
150 E. Harmon Avenue
Suite 228
Las Vegas, NV 90109

NEW JERSEY

Dennis J. Duffy
Axiom Review
33 Bleeker Street
Millburn, NJ 07042

Kathleen Passantino
Vice-President
Blue Connection
25A-288 Vreeland Road
Florham Park, NJ 07932

Marc Allen
Medical Review Corporation
237 South Street
Morristown, NJ 07906

NEW YORK

Patrick Kearse
President
Corporate Care Management
32 Broad Avenue
Binghamton, NY 13903

Theodore Will
Island Peer Review
Organization, Inc.
96-25 Queens Boulevard
10th Floor
Rego Park, NY 11374

Dr. Madelon Lubin Finkel
Chief Executive Officer
Second Opinion Consultants, Inc.
P.O. Box 621
Millwood, NY 10546

NORTH CAROLINA

Lori Carter
Medcost, Inc.
2150 Country Club Road
Suite 160
Winston-Salem, NC 27014

Dr. Richard Kevecman
President
Metrolina Medical Foundation
3000 Charlottetown Center
Charlotte, NC 28204

OHIO

John O. Micha
President
Alternative Care Management
Systems, Inc.
3539 Snouffer Road
Suite 100
Columbus, OH 43235

Janice Spillane
CoMed Management, Inc.
525 Metro Place N.
Suite 300
Dublin, OH 43017

Maribeth Harr
Comprehensive Review
Technology, Inc.
455 E. Mound Street
Columbus, OH 43215

Ginny Leitch
GreenTree Health Services, Inc.
P.O. Box 1005
Delaware, OH 43015

Maribeth Harr
Health Benefits Group, Inc.
941 Chatham Lane
Suite 103
Columbus, OH 43221

William Stief
Health Service Review, Inc.
6730 Roosevelt
Franklin, OH 45005

Warren D. Fuller
Integrated Health Systems, Inc.
119 Dillmont Drive
Worthington, OH 43085

Michael Linde
Med-Valu by MHC
6200 D Avery Road
Dublin, OH 43017

James W. Harless
Mutual Health Services Co.
1240 Huron Road
Cleveland, OH 44115

John Cannon
Peer Review Systems, Inc.
3700 Corporate Drive
Suite 250
Columbus, OH 43231

Christine Haydock, R.N.
Preview-Health Benefits
   Management of Ohio, Inc.
3737 Sylvania Avenue
Toledo, OH 43696

OKLAHOMA

Ralph S. Rhoades
Member Service Administrators
1437 S. Boulder
Tulsa, OK 74119

OREGON

Rylla Riverman, R.N.
Vice-President, Operations
ValuTrac Health Care
   Management Services
1815 S.W. Marlow
Suite 209
Portland, OR 97225

PENNSYLVANIA

Dr. Mel S. Goldsmith
Acorn PsychManagement Corp.
Robert Morris Building
17th & Arch Streets
Philadelphia, PA 18103

Jerry Boyer
Vice-President
Health Benefits Management,
   Inc./The Precertification
   Center
P.O. Box 8125
Camp Hill, PA 17089

Marilyn Morris
Health Related Services, Inc.
301 Fifth Avenue Building
Pittsburgh, PA 15322

Doris Leland
IntraCorp
1295 Westlakes Drive
Berwyn, PA 19312

Robert Bauer
Chief Executive Officer
Med-Services Management Co.
1 Bala Avenue
Suite 4C
Bala-Cynwyd, PA 19004

Joseph McCabe
President
Options—Experts in Disability
  Management
HCCC Division
400 Penn Center Boulevard
Suite 741
Pittsburgh, PA 15235

J. M. Kennedy
Quality Health Services, Inc.
633 W. Germantown Pike
Plymouth Meeting, PA 19462

Anthony Panzetta, M.D.
TAO, Inc.
P.O. Box 58655
Philadelphia, PA 19102

Cathy Baer
Universal Managed Care, Inc.
70 N. Main Street
Wilkes-Barre, PA 18711

TENNESSEE

Tim Rout
Behavioral Health Group
2693 Union Avenue Extended
Suite 101
Memphis, TN 38112

Dr. Roger Taylor
Corporate Health Care
  Management
1801 West End Avenue
P.O. Box 1115
Nashville, TN 37202

Stuart Goldstein
Focus Healthcare Management
7101 Executive Center Drive
Suite 160
Brentwood, TN 37027

Donna Miller
Memphis Business Group on
  Health
2675 Union Extended
Memphis, TN 38112

TEXAS

Frank Breaney
President
American Health Network, Inc.
3988 N. Central Expressway
Dallas, TX 75204

Stephen F. Coady
Health Economics Corp.
1300 W. Mockingbird Lane
Dallas, TX 75247

Carolyn Rich
Quality, Inc.
11498 Luna Road
Suite 103
Dallas, TX 75234

UTAH

Becky Mattingly
Health Strategies, Inc.
2610 Decker Lane
Salt Lake City, UT 84119

Diane Holye
Executive Vice-President
Medical Review Institute of
  America
525 E. 100 South
Suite 300
Salt Lake City, UT 84102

Susan Carver, R.N.
Smith Associates (SA Care)
P.O. Box 6123
Salt Lake City, UT 84106

VIRGINIA

Elizabeth Friberg
Assistant Vice-President for
  Clinical Operations
American PsychManagement,
  Inc.
1560 Wilson Boulevard
Suite 100
Arlington, VA 22209

Blue Cross/Blue Shield of
  Virginia
P.O. Box 27401
Richmond, VA 28279

Debbie L. Scheff
President
Health Cost Consultants, Inc.
10201 Lee Highway
Fairfax, VA 22030

Vivian Ward
VPS Case Management
  Services, Inc.
4335 Cox Road
Glen Allen, VA 23060

WISCONSIN

Richard Blomquist
Associates for Health Care, Inc.
150 N. Sunnyslope Road
Brookfield, WI 53005

Susan Kraus
Blue Cross/Blue Shield United of
  Wisconsin/The Advantage
  Program
401 W. Michigan Street
Milwaukee, WI 53201

Mark Williams
National Health Services Inc.
  (Care Review)
12300 W. Center Street
Milwaukee, WI 53222

CHIEF EXECUTIVE OFFICERS
OR MEDICAL DIRECTORS OF MAJOR
HEALTH INSURANCE COMPANIES

Aetna Life & Casualty
151 Farmington Avenue
Hartford, CT 06156
Howard L. Bailit, Vice-President,
Medical Management
Telephone: 203/273-0123

Combined Insurance Company of
America
123 North Wacker Drive
Chicago, IL 60606
Leonard Hertko, M.D., Medical
Director
Telephone: 312/701-3000

Connecticut General Life
Insurance Company
Employee Benefits and Health
Care Group
900 Cottage Grove Road
Bloomfield, CT 06002
Mail to: Hartford, CT 06152
G. Robert O'Brien, President
Telephone: 203/726-6000

(Continental Assurance
Company)
CNA Insurance Companies
CNA Plaza
Chicago, IL 60685
Gerald J. Foley, M.D., Vice-
President & Medical Director
Philip L. Bryson, M.D., Associate
Medical Director
Telephone: 312/822-5000

Employers Health Insurance
Company
1 WEG Boulevard
Green Bay, WI 54344
Norman Schroeder, M.D.,
Assistant Vice-President &
Medical Director
Telephone: 414/336-1100 or
800/558-4444

General American Life Insurance
  Company
700 Market Street
St. Louis, MO 63101
Mail to: P.O. Box 396
St. Louis, MO 63166
Charles B. Ladd, M.D., Medical
  Vice-President
Telephone: 314/231-1700

The Guardian Life Insurance
  Company of America
201 Park Avenue South
New York, NY 10003
Frederick E. Lewis, M.D., Second
  Vice-President & Medical
  Director
Telephone: 212/598-8000

John Hancock Mutual Life
  Insurance Company
P.O. Box 111
Boston, MA 02117
Cesar I. Gonzales, M.D., General
  Medical Director
Telephone: 617/572-6000

The Lincoln National Life
  Insurance Company
1300 South Clinton Street
Fort Wayne, IN 46801
Mail to: P.O. Box 1110
Fort Wayne, IN 46801
Ian M. Rolland, Chairman,
  President & Chief Executive
  Officer
Telephone: 219/455-2000

Massachusetts Mutual Life
  Insurance Company
1295 State Street
Springfield, MA 01111
John P. Carey, M.D., Vice-
  President & Chief Medical
  Director
Telephone: 413/788-8411

Metropolitan Life Insurance
  Company
One Madison Avenue
New York, NY 10010
William T. Friedewald, M.D.,
  Vice-President & Chief Medical
  Director
Telephone: 212/578-2211

Mutual Benefit Life Insurance
  Company
Corporate Home Office
520 Broad Street
Newark, NJ 07102-3184
Telephone: 201/481-8000
Richard Don King, M.D.,
  Vice-President & Chief
  Medical Director

Mutual of Omaha Insurance
  Company
Mutual of Omaha Plaza
Omaha, NE 68175
Kenneth L. McDonough,
  Vice-President & Medical
  Director
Telephone: 402/342-7600

New York Life Insurance
  Company
51 Madison Avenue
New York, NY 10010
John R. Iacovino, M.D.,
  Vice-President
Telephone: 212/576-7000

The Principal Financial Group
711 High Street
Des Moines, IA 50392-0001
Greg D. Haessler, M.D., Medical
  Director
Telephone: 515/247-5111

Provident Life and Accident
  Insurance Company
1 Fountain Square
Chattanooga, TN 37402
William Feist, M.D., Vice-
  President & Corporation
  Medical Director
Telephone: 615/755-1011

The Prudential Insurance
  Company of America
751 Broad Street
Newark, NJ 07102-3777
Richard Bailey, M.D., Vice-
  President & Chief Medical
  Director
Telephone: 201/802-6000

State Farm Mutual Automobile
  Insurance Company
One State Farm Plaza
Bloomington, IL 61710-0001
Dan L. Scott, M.D., Vice-
  President & Medical Director
Telephone: 309/766-2311

Time Insurance Company
501 West Michigan
Milwaukee, WI 53201
Mail to: P.O. Box 3050
Milwaukee, WI 53201-3050
Jack Lane, M.D., Medical Director
Telephone: 414/271-3011

The Travelers Insurance Company
One Tower Square
Hartford, CT 06183
David J. Ottensmeyer, M.D.,
  Senior Vice-President & Chief
  Medical Director
Telephone: 203/277-0111

United American Insurance
  Company
2909 North Buckner Boulevard
Dallas, TX 75228
Mail to: P.O. Box 810
Dallas, TX 75221-0810
Chester Cook, Medical Director
Telephone: 214/328-2841

Unum Life Insurance Company
2211 Congress Street
Portland, ME 04122
Mark E. Battista, M.D., Vice-
  President & Medical Director
Telephone: 207/770-2211

STATE INSURANCE COMMISSIONERS

Mike Weaver
Commissioner
135 South Union Street
Montgomery, Alabama 36104
Telephone: 205/269-3550
Fax: 205/240-3194

David Walsh
Director
333 Willoughby Avenue
9th Floor
P.O. Box D
Juneau, Alaska 99811-0800
Telephone: 907/465-2515
Fax: 907/463-3841

Fanene Su'a Scanlan
Commissioner
Office of the Governor
Pago Pago, American Samoa 96797
Telephone: 011-684/633-4116

Susan Gallinger
Director
3030 North 3rd Street
Suite 100
Phoenix, Arizona 85012
Telephone: 602/255-5400
Fax: 602/255-4722

Ron Taylor
Commissioner
400 University Tower Building
12th and University Streets
Little Rock, Arkansas 72204
Telephone: 501/371-1325
Fax: 501/371-5723

Roxani Gillespie
Commissioner
100 Van Ness Avenue
San Francisco, California 94102
Telephone: 415/557-9624
Fax: 415/557-3076

3450 Wilshire Boulevard
#201
Los Angeles, California 90010
Telephone: 213/736-2572
Fax: 213/736-4800

Joanne Hill
Commissioner
303 West Colfax Avenue
5th Floor
Denver, Colorado 80204
Telephone: 303/620-4300

Peter F. Kelly
Commissioner
165 Capitol Avenue
State Office Building
Hartford, Connecticut 06106
Telephone: 203/297-3801
Fax: 203/566-7410

David N. Levinson
Commissioner
Rodney Building
841 Silver Lake Boulevard
Dover, Delaware 19901
Telephone: 302/736-4251
Fax: 302/736-5280

Margurite C. Stokes
Superintendent
613 G Street, N.W.
6th Floor
Washington, DC 20001
Telephone: 202/727-7424
Fax: 202/727-7940

Tom Gallagher
Commissioner
Attn: Larry Bodkin, Assistant
   to Treasurer
State Capitol
Plaza Level Eleven
Tallahassee, Florida 32399-0300
Telephone: 904/488-3440
Fax: 904/488-6581

Warren D. Evans
Commissioner
2 Martin L. King, Jr., Drive
Floyd Memorial Building
704 West Tower
Atlanta, Georgia 30334
Telephone: 404/656-2056

Joaquin G. Blaz
Commissioner
855 West Marine Drive
Agana, Guam 96910
Telephone: 011-671/477-5106
Fax: 011-671/472-2643

Robin Campaniano
1010 Richards Street
Honolulu, Hawaii 96813
Telephone: 808/548-5450
Fax: 808/543-2721

Tony Fagiano
Director
500 South 10th Street
Boise, Idaho 83720
Telephone: 208/334-2250
Fax: 208/334-2298

State of Illinois Center
100 W. Randolph Street
Suite 15-100
Chicago, Illinois 60601
Telephone: 312/917-2420
Fax: 312/917-5435

Zack Stamp
Director
320 West Washington Street
4th Floor
Springfield, Illinois 62767
Telephone: 217/782-4515
Fax: 217/782-5020

John J. Dillon III
Commissioner
311 West Washington Street
Suite 300
Indianapolis, Indiana 46204-2787
Telephone: 317/232-2385
Fax: 317/237-4949

Lucas State Office Building
6th Floor
Des Moines, Iowa 50319
Telephone: 515/281-5705
Fax: 515/281-3059

Fletcher Bell
Commissioner
420 S.W. 9th Street
Topeka, Kansas 66612
Telephone: 913/296-7801
Fax: 913/296-2283

Elizabeth P. Wright
Commissioner
229 West Main Street
Frankfort, Kentucky 40602
Telephone: 502/564-3630
Fax: 502/564-6090

Douglas D. Green
Commissioner
950 North 5th Street
Baton Rouge, Louisiana 70801-9214
Telephone: 504/342-5900
Fax: 504/342-3078

Joseph A. Edwards
Superintendent
State Office Building
State House, Station 34
Augusta, Maine 04333
Telephone: 207/582-8707
Fax: 207/582-8716

John A. Donaho
Commissioner
501 St. Paul Place
Stanbalt Building
7th Floor - South
Baltimore, Maryland 21202
Telephone: 410/333-2520
Fax: 410/333-1229

Timothy H. Gailey
Commissioner
280 Friend Street
Boston, Massachusetts 02114
Telephone: 617/727-7189
Fax: 617/727-7189/ext. 299

Dhiraj Shah
Acting Commissioner
611 West Ottawa Street
2nd Floor North
Lansing, Michigan 48933
Telephone: 517/373-9273
Fax: 517/335-4978

Thomas H. Borman
Commissioner
133 East 7th Street
St. Paul, Minnesota 55101
Telephone: 612/296-6848
Fax: 612/296-4328

George Dale
Commissioner
1804 Walter Sillers Building
Jackson, Mississippi 39205
Telephone: 601/359-3569
Fax: 601/359-2474

Lewis Melahn
Director
301 West High Street 6 North
Jefferson City, Missouri 65102-0690
Telephone: 314/751-4126
Fax: 314/751-1165

Andrea Bennett
Commissioner
126 North Sanders
Mitchell Building, Room 270
Helena, Montana 59601
Telephone: 406/444-2040
Fax: 406/444-3497

William H. McCartney
Director
Terminal Building
941 'O' Street
Suite 400
Lincoln, Nebraska 68508
Telephone: 402/471-2201
Fax: 402/471-4610

Al Iuppa
Commissioner
1665 Hot Springs Road
Carson City, Nevada 89710
Telephone: 702/687-4270
Fax: 702/687-3937

Louis E. Bergeron
Commissioner
169 Manchester Street
Concord, New Hampshire 03301
Telephone: 603/271-2261
Fax: 603/271-1406

Samuel F. Fortunato
Commissioner
20 West State Street CN325
Trenton, New Jersey 08625
Telephone: 609/292-5363
Fax: 609/633-3601

Fabian Chavez
Superintendent
P.O. Drawer 1269
Sante Fe, New Mexico 87504-1269
Telephone: 505/827-4500
Fax: 505/827-4734

Salvtore R. Curiale
Superintendent
160 West Broadway
New York, New York 10013
Telephone: 212/602-0429
Fax: 212/602-0437

James E. Long
Commissioner
Dobbs Building
430 Salisbury Street
Raleigh, North Carolina 27611
Telephone: 919/733-7349
Fax: 919/733-6495

Earl R. Pomeroy
Commissioner
600 E. Boulevard
Bismarck, North Dakota 58505-
0320
Telephone: 701/224-2440
Fax: 701/224-4880

George Fabe
Director
2100 Stella Court
Columbus, Ohio 43266-0566
Telephone: 614/644-2658

Gerald Grimes
Commissioner
1901 North Walnut
Oklahoma City, Oklahoma 73105
Telephone: 405/521-2828
Fax: 405/521-6652

Theodore R. Kulongoski
Commissioner
21 Labor and Industries Building
Salem, Oregon 97310
Telephone: 503/378-4271
Fax: 503/378-4351

Constance B. Foster
Commissioner
Strawberry Square
13th Floor
Harrisburg, Pennsylvania 17120
Telephone: 717/787-5173
Fax: 717/783-1059

Miguel A. Villafane
Commissioner
Fernandez Juncos Station
1607 Ponce De Leon Avenue
Santurce, Puerto Rico 00910
Telephone: 809/722-8686
Fax: 809/722-4400

Robert J. Janes
Commissioner
233 Richmond Street
Suite 237
Providence, Rhode Island 02903-
4237
Telephone: 401/277-2246

John G. Richards
Commissioner
1612 Marion Street
Columbia, South Carolina 29201
Telephone: 803/737-6205
Fax: 803/737-6205

Mary Jane Cleary
Director
Insurance Building
910 E. Sioux Avenue
Pierre, South Dakota 57501
Telephone: 605/773-3563
Fax: 605/773-5369

Elaine A. McReynolds
Commissioner
Volunteer Plaza
500 James Robertson Parkway
Nashville, Tennessee 37219
Telephone: 615/741-2241
Fax: 615/741-4000

Jo Ann Howard
Board Member
1110 San Jacinto Boulevard
Austin, Texas 78701-1998
Telephone: 512/463-6332
Fax: 512/463-0866

Richard F. Reynolds
Board Member
1110 San Jacinto Boulevard
Austin, Texas 78701-1998
Telephone: 512/463-9979
Fax: 512/463-0866

James E. Saxton, Jr.
Chairman—State Board
1110 San Jacinto Boulevard
Austin, Texas 78701-1998
Telephone: 512/463-6330
Fax: 512/463-0866

A. W. Pogue
Commissioner
1110 San Jacinto Boulevard
Austin, Texas 78701-1998
Telephone: 512/463-6464
Fax: 512/475-2005

Harold C. Yancey
Commissioner
3110 State Office Building
Salt Lake City, Utah 84114-1201
Telephone: 801/538-3800
Fax: 801/538-3829

Jeffrey Johnson
Commissioner
State Office Building
Montpelier, Vermont 05602
Telephone: 802/828-3301
Fax: 802/828-3306

Steven T. Foster
Commissioner
1220 Jefferson Building
1220 Bank Street
Richmond, Virginia 23219
Telephone: 804/786-3741
Fax: 804/786-3396

Derek M. Hodge
Commissioner
Kongens Gade #18
Saint Thomas, Virgin Islands
  00802
Telephone: 809/774-2991
Fax: 809/774-6953

Richard G. Marquardt
Commissioner
Insurance Building AQ21
Olympia, Washington 98504
Telephone: 206/753-7301
Fax: 206/586-3535

Hanley C. Clark
Commissioner
2019 Washington Street East
Charleston, West Virginia 25305
Telephone: 304/348-3394
Fax: 304/438-0412

Robert D. Haase
Commissioner
121 East Wilson
Madison, Wisconsin 53702
Telephone: 608/266-0102
Fax: 608/266-9935

Kenneth Erickson
Commissioner
Herschler Building
122 West 25th Street
Cheyenne, Wyoming 82002
Telephone: 307/777-7401
Fax: 307/777-5895

SELECTED BIBLIOGRAPHY

MANAGED CARE

American Psychiatric Association: Manual of Psychiatric Quality Assurance. Washington, DC, American Psychiatric Association, 1992

Bably N, Sullivan S: Buying Smart: Business Strategies for Managing Health Care Costs. Washington, DC, American Enterprise Institute, 1986

Berenson RA: A physician's perspective on case management. Business and Health 2(8):22–25, 1985

Boland P (ed): Making Managed Care Work: A Practical Guide to Strategies and Solutions. New York, McGraw-Hill, 1990

Bridwell D, Collins J, Levine D: A quiet revolution: the movement of EAPs to managed care. EAP Digest 8:27–30, 1988

Capron AM: Containing health care costs: ethical and legal implications of changes in the methods of paying physicians. Case Western Reserve Law Review 36:708–759, 1986

Cowan D: Preferred Provider Organizations. Rockville, MD, Aspen, 1984

Donabedian A: The Definition of Quality and Approaches to Its Assessment. Ann Arbor, MI, Health Administration Press, 1980

Donabedian A: Explorations in Quality Assessment and Monitoring: The Criteria and Standards of Quality. Ann Arbor, MI, Health Administration Press, 1982

Ferlstrein P, Wickizer T, Wheeler J: Private cost containment: the effects of utilization review programs on health care use and expenditures. N Engl J Med 318:1310–1314, 1988

Fielding JE: Corporate Health Management. Menlo Park, CA, Addison-Wesley, 1984

Fox P: Synthesis of Private Sector Health Care Initiatives (Contract No HHS 100-82-0031). Washington, DC, Office of Assistant Secretary for Planning and Evaluation, U.S. Department of Health and Human Services, March 1984

Fox P, Goldbeck W, Spres F: Health Care Cost Management. Ann Arbor, MI, Health Administration Press, 1984

Frank R, Salkever D: Report on Expenditure and Utilization Patterns for Mental Illness and Substance Abuse Services. Baltimore, MD, Johns Hopkins University, 1990

Frank R, Salkever D, Sharfstein S: A new look at rising mental health insurance costs. Health Affairs, Summer 1991, pp 116–123

Furrow BR: The ethics of cost-containment: bureaucratic medicine and doctors as patient advocate. Notre Dame Journal of Law, Ethics and Public Policy 3:187–225, 1988

Goldstein J, Horgan C: Inpatient and outpatient psychiatric services: substitutes or complements? Hosp Community Psychiatry 39:632–636, 1988

Hamilton J (ed): Psychiatric Peer Review—Prelude and Promise. Washington, DC, American Psychiatric Press, 1985

Institute of Medicine: Controlling Costs and Changing Patient Care: The Role of Utilization Management. Washington, DC, National Academy Press, 1989

Joint Commission on Accreditation of Hospitals: Accreditation Manual for Hospitals. Chicago, IL, Joint Commission on Accreditation of Hospitals, 1985

Kessler L, Steinwachs D, Hankin J: Episodes of psychiatric care and mental utilization. Med Care 20:1209–1221, 1982

Kiesler C: Public and professional myths about mental hospitalization: an empirical reassessment of policy-related beliefs. Am Psychol 37:1323–1339, 1982

Kiesler C, Sibulkin A: Mental Hospitalization: Myths and Facts About a National Crisis. Newbury Park, CA, Sage, 1987

Kongstavedt P: The Managed Health Care Handbook. Rockville, MD, Aspen, 1989

London P, Klerman HL: Evaluating psychotherapy. Am J Psychiatry 139:709–717, 1982

MacKenzie K: Recent developments in brief psychotherapy. Hosp Community Psychiatry 39:742–752, 1988

Mechanic D: Cost containment and the quality of medical care: rationing strategies in an era of constrained resources. Milbank Memorial Fund Quarterly: Health and Society 63:453–475, 1985

Melnick S, Lyter L: The negative impacts of increased concurrent review of psychiatric inpatient care. Hosp Community Psychiatry 38:300–302, 1987

Miller W, Hester R: Inpatient alcoholism treatment: who benefits? Am Psychol 41:794–805, 1986

Milstein A, Oehm M, Alpert G: Gauging the performance of utilization review. Business and Health 4:10–12, 1987

National Association of Private Psychiatric Hospitals: Ensuring Good Psychiatric Benefits. Washington, DC, National Association of Private Psychiatric Hospitals, 1988

National Health Lawyer's Association: The Insider's Guide to Managed Care: A Legal and Operational Roadmap. Washington, DC, National Health Lawyer's Association, 1990

Parloff MB: Psychotherapy research evidence and reimbursement decisions. Am J Psychiatry 139:718–727, 1982

Perlman BB, Melnick D, Kentera A: Assessing the effectiveness of a case management program. Hosp Community Psychiatry 36:405–407, 1985

Povar G, Moreno J: Hippocrates and the health maintenance organization. Ann Intern Med 109:419–424, 1988

Reagan MD: Physicians as gatekeepers: a complex challenge. N Engl J Med 1731–1734, 1987

Rodriguez AR: Current and future direction in reimbursement for psychiatric services. Gen Hosp Psychiatry 7:341–348, 1985

The Effects of Contemporary Economic Conditions on Availability and Quality of Mental Health Services. New York, Plenum, 1987

Sanazarro PJ: Quality Assessment and Quality Assurance in Medical Care (Annual Review of Public Health: Volume I, Breslow L, ed). Palo Alto, CA, Annual Reviews, 1980

Schacht TE, Strupp HH: Evaluation of psychotherapy, in Comprehensive Textbook of Psychiatry/IV, 4th Edition. Edited by Kaplan HI, Sadock BJ. Baltimore, MD, Williams & Wilkins, 1985

Sharfstein SS, Beigel A (eds): The New Economics and Psychiatric Care. Washington, DC, American Psychiatric Press, 1985

Sharfstein SS, Patterson DY: The growing crisis in access to mental health services for middle-class families. Am J Psychiatry 34:1009–1014, 1983

Sharfstein SS, Taube CA: Reductions in insurance for mental disorders: adverse selection, moral hazard and consumer demand. Am J Psychiatry 139:1425–1430, 1982

Steffen G: Quality medical care. JAMA 260:56–61, 1988

Tischler G: Utilization management of mental health services by private third parties. Am J Psychiatry 147:967–973, 1990

Trauner J: The next generation of utilization review. Business and Health 4:14–16, 1987

Williamson JW, Hudson JI, Nevins WW: Principles of Quality Assurance and Cost Containment in Health Care. San Francisco, CA, Jossey-Bass, 1982

EFFECTIVENESS OF PSYCHIATRIC CARE

American Medical Association, Council on Long Range Planning and Development: The future of psychiatry. JAMA 264:2549–2556, 1990

American Psychiatric Association: Treatments of Psychiatric Disorders: A Task Force Report of the American Psychiatric Association. Washington, DC, American Psychiatric Association, 1989

Frank E, Kupfer DJ, Perel JM, et al: Three-year outcomes for maintenance therapies in recurrent depression. Arch Gen Psychiatry 47:1093–1099, 1990

Office of Technology Assessment: Implications of Cost-Effectiveness Analysis of Medical Technology No 3: The Efficacy and Cost-Effectiveness of Psychotherapy. Washington, DC, Office of Technology Assessment, 1980

Parloff M: Assessment of psychosocial treatment of mental health disorders. Report to the National Academy of Sciences, Institute of Medicine, Washington, DC, 1978

Sharfstein S, Magnas H: Insuring intensive psychotherapy. Am J Psychiatry 132:1252–1256, 1975

Smith M, Glass G, Miller T: The Benefits of Psychotherapy. Baltimore, MD, Johns Hopkins University Press, 1980

Wells K: The Functioning and Well-Being of Depressed Patients: Results From the Medical Outcome Study. Santa Monica, CA, Rand, 1989

COST OFFSET OF PSYCHIATRIC CARE

Department of Health and Human Services: Report of the Alcohol, Drug and Mental Health Administration Primary Work Group. Washington, DC, Department of Health and Human Services, 1985

Follette WT, Cummings NA: Psychiatric services and medical utilization in a prepaid health plan setting. Med Care 5:25–35, 1967

Jones KR, Vischi TR: Impact of alcohol, drug abuse and mental health treatment on medical care utilization: a review of the research literature. Med Care 17 (suppl 12), 1979

Mumford E, Schlesinger H, Glass G, et al: A new look at evidence about reduced cost of medical utilization following mental health treatment. Am J Psychiatry 141:1145–1156, 1984

Sharfstein S, Magnas H: Insuring intensive psychotherapy. Am J Psychiatry 132:1252–1256, 1975